THE ULTIMATE METABOLIC CONFUSION DIET FOR ENDOMORPH WOMEN

This guide offers a balanced diet with a meal plan and tasty recipes for weight loss, metabolism activation, and fitness goal achievement from breakfast to dinner.

Vincent John Walker

Disclaimer

This publication is designed to provide competent and reliable information regarding the subject covered. However, the views expressed in this publication are those of the author alone, and should not be taken as expert instruction or professional advice. The reader is responsible for his or her actions. The author hereby disclaims any responsibility or liability whatsoever that is incurred from the use or application of the contents of this publication by the purchaser of the reader. The purchaser or reader is hereby responsible for his or her actions.

Copyright © 2024

Table of Contents

INTRODUCTION

"Metabolic Confusion" is a notion that has gained favor in recent years as a novel method for weight control and general metabolic health. This technique helps individuals achieve a healthier metabolism. It entails introducing modifications in both your food and exercise habits in a smart manner to prevent your body from becoming used to a certain pattern.

In its most basic form, metabolic confusion is an attempt to prevent the body from falling into a pattern that might result in a halt in either the rate of weight loss or the acceleration of muscle building. The fundamental concept is that you might increase your metabolism and accomplish more consistent success over time if you avoid doing things in a constant pattern and keep your body guessing about what you are doing.

The concept of metabolic confusion may be used in a variety of contexts:

Altering the amount of macronutrients you consume and the number of calories you consume at various intervals is what is meant by the term "dietary variation." To give you an example, you could have days when you consume more carbohydrates than usual, followed by days when you consume less. It is considered that this variation helps to maintain an active and adaptive metabolism when observed.

Changing your total calorie intake is the goal of the caloric cycling strategy, which is analogous to adjusting the amount of macronutrients you consume. Your calorie intake may fluctuate from day to day, with some days having a higher calorie intake than others. This volatility is supposed to prevent your body from adapting to a stable calorie count, which would otherwise be the case.

Intermittent Fasting: Another aspect of metabolic confusion is the incorporation of patterns of intermittent fasting. Altering the time of your meals and periods of fasting may affect how your body consumes energy and how it regulates fat.

The metabolic confusion extends to your training regimen, therefore it's important to vary your exercises. You would include a variety of distinct sorts of workouts, such as high-intensity interval training (HIIT), strength training, and cardiovascular exercise, rather than keeping to the same activities and intensity levels throughout your workout routine.

Altering the time and frequency of meals and exercises is another component of metabolic confusion. Altering the schedule of meals and workouts may also be difficult. Altering some aspects of your routine, such as the time you work out or the frequency of your meals, may bring an element of unpredictability to your routine.

It should be brought to your attention that metabolic confusion, even though it is an interesting approach, is not a universally applicable solution.

People who have reached a point in their effort to lose weight when they have reached a plateau or who are looking to reinvigorate their fitness progress may find that metabolic confusion is especially appealing. On the other hand, just like any other aspect of your lifestyle, it must be adapted to your requirements and tastes.

Advantages of Metabolic Confusion

Metabolic confusion offers many potential advantages, which have led to its popularity as a weight reduction and fitness strategy. Here is a list of some of the primary benefits:

- Plateau Avoidance: Metabolic confusion makes it harder for the body to adapt to a new diet or exercise regimen.
- You may be able to avoid the weight loss or muscle-building plateaus that are common with continuous routines if you prevent adaptation.
- Increased Metabolic Flexibility: The approach assists the body in becoming metabolically flexible, which means it can efficiently transition between utilizing carbohydrates and fats for energy.
- This adaptation has the potential to boost fat metabolism and total energy expenditure.

- Constant Calorie Burn: Changing up your diet and workout routine might help keep your metabolism going.

- This might lead to a consistent calorie expenditure throughout the day, even while you're sleeping.

- Increased Fat Loss: Metabolic confusion may increase fat loss by preventing the body from adapting to a particular calorie intake or macronutrient distribution.

- Because of the constantly changing environment, the body may become increasingly reliant on stored fat for energy.

- Muscle Retention: Varying your exercises and intensity levels will help you prevent muscle adaptation and breakdown.

- This is particularly important while attempting to reduce weight since muscular mass encourages a quicker metabolic rate.

- Increased Fitness Progress: The approach may result in increases in strength, endurance, and overall fitness.

- Variable workouts put diverse muscle groups and energy systems to the test, which leads to overall fitness progress.

- Psychological Participation: Metabolic ambiguity makes your routine interesting and new.

- Trying different routines, altering your nutrition, and embracing change may assist you in avoiding boredom and remaining motivated.

- Adaptable to Individual Preferences: Metabolic confusion may be customized to different eating patterns and fitness levels.

- It is versatile and may be adapted to each individual's requirements.

- Potential Hormonal Benefits: Altering between caloric deficit and maintenance periods may assist in minimizing hormonal imbalances that might occur with long-term calorie restriction.

- This may help to maintain balanced hormone levels, which are necessary for overall health.

- Long-term viability: The strategy promotes a way of life that is free of strict and monotonous routines.

- This may result in a long-term, sustainable way of eating and exercising.

- Breaking Through Weight Loss Stagnation: Metabolic confusion is particularly advantageous for persons who have hit weight loss plateaus since it gives new components to re-start progress.

- Individual aims, hobbies, and lifestyles may all be accommodated via metabolic confusion.

Personalization boosts the likelihood of success and long-term adherence.

Endomorph Women and the Metabolic Confusion Approach

Adapting the Metabolic Confusion technique for endomorph women entails tailoring the strategy to their requirements. Endomorphs are more likely to have greater body fat and a slower metabolism, which may make weight management more difficult. The following are some tips for making the Metabolic Confusion technique work successfully for endomorph women:

- Eat Healthy Meals: Focus on eating foods that are nutritious and excellent for you.

- Choose meals that are high in complex carbohydrates, lean proteins, and healthy fats.

- Modify Your Diet: Keep track of how many calories you consume, particularly because endomorphs tend to acquire weight more readily.

- To keep your body guessing, alternate between eating more and eating less.

- Vary Your Nutrients: Alter your carbohydrate, protein, and fat intake, but make sure you receive enough protein.

- Eat more carbohydrates some days and less others, so your body does not get used to a certain routine.

- Get Stronger: Perform strength training activities regularly to increase and maintain muscular strength.

- Muscles serve to increase your metabolism and offer you a more toned appearance.

- Experiment with Different Exercises: Perform both steady and vigorous workouts, such as rapid bursts of strenuous activity.

- Intense exercises might help you burn calories even after you stop working out.

- Consider When You Eat: Intermittent fasting may be a fantastic idea, but make sure it works for you.

- Eat at some times and fast at others, but make sure you receive enough nutrition.

- Watch Your Carbohydrates: Watch your carbs, particularly sugary and simple carbs.

- For long-lasting energy, choose healthy grains, veggies, and fruits.

- Consume Enough Protein: Protein promotes muscle growth and repair, which is especially crucial for endomorphs.

- To feel full and keep your muscles strong, consume lean protein with each meal.

- Mind Your Portion Quantities: Because endomorphs tend to accumulate additional fat, keep your portion sizes in control.

- Even if the meal is nutritious, be sure you're not consuming too much.

- Be Patient and Keep Going: It's important to stick to your strategy and be persistent, even if you don't notice significant results immediately.

- Endomorphs may need to wait a little longer to see benefits, but don't give up!

- Drink Water and Sleep: To boost your metabolism and general health, stay hydrated and get adequate sleep.

- Pay Attention to Your Body: Pay attention to how your body responds to certain diets and workouts.

- Adjust your strategy depending on how you feel and what works for you.

How This Book Can Help You

This book is a comprehensive guide to understanding, executing, and succeeding with the metabolic confusion strategy, which was created specifically for endomorph women. Here are some examples of how the book might assist you:

- **Understanding Metabolic Confusion:** The book starts with a definition of metabolic confusion, its benefits, and how it may be adjusted to endomorph women. This is the foundation for your future education.

- **Endomorph Body Types:** You'll get a complete understanding of endomorph body types, including their characteristics and issues. This comprehension allows you to specify your individual needs.

- **Metabolic Confusion Science:** You will study metabolism and why the metabolic confusion approach works for endomorphs. This comprehension explains the "why" underlying the strategy.

- **The basic concepts of the Metabolic Confusion Diet** are described in this chapter, including macronutrient cycling and calorie variation. You'll learn how to apply these ideas to your eating habits.

- **Making Your Metabolic Confusion Meal Plan:** The book leads you through the process of developing a personalized meal plan based on metabolic confusion ideas. Sample meal plans adapted to different calorie needs can assist you in getting started.

- **Implementing Metabolic Confusion Activities:** You will learn how to organize your exercises to maximize the metabolic confusion impact. To keep your body responsive, the chapter addresses how to include strength training, HIIT, and other exercises into your regimen.

- **Overcoming Obstacles and Maintaining Consistency:** In this chapter, we'll talk about common hurdles including cravings and emotional eating. There are several methods for maintaining consistency in social environments. This guidance will help you stay on track in real-world situations.

- **Recipes & Meal Prep for Success:** Practical meal prep advice and a wide range of healthy dishes save you time and help you meet your nutritional goals. Grocery shopping and culinary skills can make meal planning simpler.

- **Listening to Your Body:** Adjustments and Plateaus: Learn to interpret your body's signals and make the necessary changes. Breaking through plateaus tactics ensures that your progress is constant.

- **Beyond the Diet:** This chapter emphasizes the need for a comprehensive approach that includes stress management, sleep, and a positive mindset. You'll be ready to make long-term changes.

Understanding Endomorph Body Types

Discovering Different Body Types

There are three basic body types, also known as somatotypes, that explain overall physical features and inclinations connected to metabolism and body composition. Ectomorph, mesomorph, and endomorph are the three body kinds. Each bodily type has various characteristics and characteristics. Here's a detailed description of each:

Ectomorph: Ectomorphs are distinguished by their slim and slender physique. They have specific distinguishing characteristics that contribute to their particular body composition and metabolism.

- *Ectomorphs often have a thin bone structure*, which is reflected in their small wrists, ankles, and shoulders. They often have a delicate, elongated frame with minimal body fat.

- *Metabolism and Weight Management:* Ectomorphs have a quick metabolism, which means their bodies burn calories quickly. This makes it difficult for them to acquire weight, especially muscular mass. Despite their attempts to increase calorie intake, ectomorphs may struggle to gain muscle.

- While ectomorphs may struggle to acquire muscle, their body type frequently allows them to retain a sleek and defined look even with no activity. Building considerable muscle mass, on the other hand, may need constant strength training and a greater calorie intake.

Mesomorph: Mesomorphs have a naturally athletic and muscular build. They have characteristics that make them ideal for athletic activity and muscular growth.

- *Physique Shape:* Mesomorphs have a well-proportioned body with a balanced bone structure. They often have a naturally athletic look, with wide shoulders, a thin waist, and visible muscular definition.

- *Muscular and Strength:* One of the most distinguishing characteristics of mesomorphs is their ability to grow muscle mass quickly. Their bodies react well to strength training and they have obvious muscular definition even when they don't exercise much.

- *Metabolism and Weight Control:* Mesomorphs have a moderate metabolism, which allows them to control their weight more readily than endomorphs. With the right diet and exercise plans, they may grow muscle and decrease fat.

Endomorph: Endomorphs have a softer and rounder body type. They have traits that determine their body composition as well as how they react to food and exercise.

- *Endomorphs often have a broader bone structure and a rounder overall look.* When compared to ectomorphs and mesomorphs, they may have a broader face and a larger proportion of body fat.

- *Metabolism and Weight Management:* Endomorphs often have a slower metabolism, which may make losing weight and maintaining a lean body more difficult. They are more prone to storing fat, particularly around the belly, hips, and thighs.

- *Endomorphs may find it simpler to build both muscle and fat,* but it is critical for them to carefully regulate their calorie intake and pick proper exercise routines to achieve a balance between muscle growth and fat removal.

Endomorph Women's Characteristics: Challenges and Strengths

Endomorph women have unique physical and metabolic traits that impact their body composition, diet and exercise response, and general health. The following are some of the qualities, problems, and strengths that are typically linked with endomorph body types:

Endomorph Women's Body Shape and Composition: Endomorph women often have a soft and curvaceous body shape. They often have a rounder look, with a broader waist, bigger hips, and a lot of body fat.

- **Fat Distribution:** Endomorphs are distinguished by their tendency to accumulate fat. This fat deposition occurs largely around the lower belly, hips, and thighs, giving to their distinctive curves.

- **Muscle Definition:** Endomorph women may have less prominent muscle definition than other body types due to a greater body fat percentage. Under the layer of stored fat, muscles may be less noticeable.

- Endomorphs often have a strong bone structure with wider shoulders and hips. This sturdy frame contributes to their more substantial look.

- **Weight Management Difficulties:** Endomorph women have weight management difficulties owing to their slower metabolic rate and propensity to accumulate fat. Weight reduction may need more work than in other body types.

Endomorph Women Face the Following Obstacles:

- **Weight Management and Fat Loss:** One of the most difficult problems is the effort to control one's weight, particularly fat. The body's tendency to accumulate fat might make reducing extra weight more difficult.

- **Fat Loss Difficulty:** Endomorphs often struggle to lose body fat and obtain a lean physique. Their bodies prefer to store fat reserves, making weight reduction attempts more difficult.

- **Balance Muscle Gain:** While endomorphs may efficiently create muscle, increasing muscle mass may result in some fat gain owing to the body's proclivity to store energy.

Endomorphs have a slower metabolic rate, which may make weight control difficult. It means they burn fewer calories, perhaps making weight reduction more difficult.

Endomorph Women Have the Following Strengths:

- *Endomorph women have an edge in terms of muscular growth, notwithstanding the obstacles.* Resistance exercise works well for their bodies, helping them to grow powerful, well-defined muscles.

- *Endomorphs' robust bone structure and increased muscle potential may result in amazing strength and power.* They often thrive in activities that require physical strength, such as weightlifting or athletics.

- *Satiety and Appetite Control:* A combination of muscle mass potential and increased body fat might result in increased sensations of fullness after meals. This might help with appetite management.

- *Endomorphs may accomplish extraordinary fitness development via constant work.* Their bodies respond well to strength training, resulting in visible gains in muscle definition and general fitness.

- *Energy Resilience:* The body's proclivity to accumulate fat may be used to preserve energy reserves. This characteristic may be useful in circumstances when food is scarce.

The Genetic Influence on Body Composition and Weight Management

Genetics has a significant impact on establishing an individual's body composition and how their body reacts to weight-management attempts. Here's a more in-depth look at the role of genetics in various areas:

Body Composition: Genetic factors have an impact on various elements of body composition, including:

- **Body Fat Distribution:** Genetics has a key role in where the body stores fat. Some individuals naturally store fat around their belly (the "apple" form), while others store it in their hips and thighs (the "pear" shape).

- **Muscular Mass Potential:** Genetic predisposition influences how easily someone can acquire and retain muscle mass. Certain people are genetically predisposed to muscular growth.

- **Your basal metabolic rate (BMR),** or the rate at which your body burns calories at rest, has a hereditary component. Certain people have a naturally higher BMR, resulting in more calories expended even when they are inactive.

- **Body Typing:** Genetic factors influence the classification of body types such as ectomorphs, mesomorphs, and endomorphs. This categorization influences natural physique, proclivity to grow muscle or store fat, and general metabolic characteristics.

Weight Management: Genetics also influence how your body responds to weight loss efforts:

- **Weight Set Point:** Your body's optimal weight range may be dictated by genetics, which is sometimes referred to as the weight set point. Your body may resist leaving this zone, making it difficult to sustain major weight changes.

- **Appetite Regulation:** How the body controls appetite and fullness is influenced by genetic factors. Some people may feel stronger hunger signals, making controlling food intake extremely difficult.

- **Hormones and Fat Storage:** Genetic differences influence the body's reactions to hormones that regulate hunger and fat storage, such as insulin and leptin.

- **Dietary Response:** Depending on one's genetic composition, one may respond differently to various diets. For example, some people may lose weight more effectively on a low-carb diet than on a balanced one.

- **Exercise Influence:** Genetics also have a part in how the body adapts to exercise. Due to genetic predispositions, certain people may experience faster muscle development or fat reduction while participating in various forms of exercise.

The Interaction of Genetics and Environment:

It's critical to understand how genetics and environment interact, including factors like food, physical exercise, and lifestyle choices:

While genetic composition stays constant, lifestyle decisions may alter how certain genes are expressed. Epigenetics is the name given to this intriguing area.

Environment Adaptation: The body adapts to its surroundings. While genetics may lead you to accumulate fat, living a healthy lifestyle might help minimize this propensity.

Individualization of Strategies:

Understanding your genetic tendencies might help you develop personalized weight-management strategies. Although genetics are important, lifestyle choices such as nutrition, exercise, sleep, and stress management are under your control and may have a substantial influence on your health and weight.

Genetics has a significant impact on body composition, weight control, and how the body reacts to various therapies. While genetic composition cannot be changed, making educated choices may improve your health and well-being. Working with healthcare specialists or registered dietitians may help you develop a personalized plan that takes your genetics and personal requirements into consideration.

The Science of Metabolic Confusion

Metabolism Explained: How Does Your Body Burn Calories?

Calorie expenditure, often known as energy expenditure, is a complicated and ongoing physiological process that happens inside the human body. The following is a summary of how your body burns calories:

BMR (Basal Metabolic Rate):

Consider your body to be a bustling factory that never shuts down, even while you're sleeping or sitting calmly. This factory, your body, requires energy to keep all of its machinery working. This is referred to as the Basal Metabolic Rate (BMR). It is the energy that your body utilizes to perform basic functions such as breathing, keeping your heart beating, producing new cells, and maintaining a comfortable body temperature. Calories are used to measure this energy. Your age, gender, weight, height, and even your genes all influence how many calories your body needs merely to survive and operate.

Physical Exercise:

Consider each movement you make as an additional chance for your body to burn calories. You use energy when you walk, run, play sports, or simply dance around your room. This is known as physical activity, and it occurs in three varieties:

- *Non-Exercise Activity Thermogenesis (NEAT):* This is a fancy word for the energy you expend while you aren't exercising but instead performing everyday activities like strolling to the shop, standing up, or tapping your foot.

- *Exercise Activity:* These are scheduled activities in which you move your body consciously, such as going for a bike ride, performing yoga, or lifting weights at the gym. The more calories you burn, the harder and longer you exercise.

- *Thermic Effect of Food (TEF):* Eating is more than simply eating great food. Your body expends energy digesting and processing the food you consume. This is referred to as the Thermic Effect of Food (TEF). Some nutrients, such as protein-rich foods, force your body to work harder to metabolize them, using more energy in the process.

Thermogenesis Adaptive:

Assume you're outside in the cold and your body begins to shiver to stay warm. This shivering is your body's method of burning more calories to generate heat. This is known as adaptive thermogenesis, and it occurs when your body uses extra energy to adjust to changes in temperature or conditions.

Hormonal Control:

Hormones are small messengers found throughout the body. These hormones influence how your body utilizes energy. Thyroid hormones, for example, operate as traffic lights, instructing your body how quickly to burn calories. Adrenaline is generated when you are worried or enthusiastic, which increases calorie burning, particularly if you are doing anything physical.

Muscle Size:

Consider your muscles to be little calorie-burning engines. The greater your muscular mass, the more energy your body needs to keep those engines working. This implies that having greater muscle mass may help you burn more calories even if you aren't moving around much.

Genetic Variables:

Your genes impact how your body burns calories in the same way that you acquire features like eye color from your parents. Some people are blessed with genes that increase their BMR, causing their bodies to burn calories more quickly. Others may have genes that predispose them to be more active.

Simply said, your body is an incredible energy-burning mechanism. Whether you're sleeping, jogging, or just eating, you're burning calories in a variety of ways. You may harness the power of calorie burning to maintain excellent health and reach your wellness objectives by knowing how these processes function and making educated decisions regarding diet, activity, and lifestyle.

What Causes Metabolic Confusion?

Metabolic confusion is a diet and exercise strategy that tries to keep one's metabolism flexible and adaptable. The strategy comprises altering one's calorie intake, macronutrient distribution, and level of physical exercise to prevent the body from adapting to a certain routine. The goal of this strategy is to optimize body fat loss, build muscle mass, and improve overall metabolic efficiency. The following is how metabolic confusion works:

- *Caloric Fluctuation:* The idea of metabolic confusion requires changing one's calorie intake regularly. Caloric intake varies by day, with some days showing greater consumption and others showing lower consumption. This phenomenon makes it difficult for the body to adjust to a consistent calorie intake, resulting in a standstill metabolic rate. By avoiding the slowing of metabolic rate caused by prolonged caloric restriction, calorie diversity promotes metabolic activity and adipose tissue decrease.

- *Macronutrient Cycling:* Similar to caloric fluctuation, metabolic confusion involves the adjustment of macronutrient allocation (carbohydrates, proteins, and lipids) within one's dietary routine. At certain times, people may wish to increase their carbohydrate intake, while at others, they may want to increase their protein intake. This approach stops the body from becoming proficient in metabolizing a certain nutrient, hence increasing nutrition utilization efficiency.

- *Intermittent fasting or meal timing:* The notion of metabolic confusion includes the use of intermittent fasting or meal timing manipulation. Intermittent fasting is a nutritional strategy that involves alternating periods of eating and fasting. This pattern may cause changes in calorie expenditure and alter insulin sensitivity, thereby enhancing fat loss and improving metabolic flexibility.

- *Exercise Variability:* The exercise component of metabolic confusion stresses the modification of physical activity intensity, duration, and mode. Various forms of exercise are alternated, including High-Intensity Interval Training (HIIT), strength training, and cardiovascular exercises. This condition impairs the body's capacity to adapt to a specific training routine, leading to increased adipose tissue loss, increased muscular growth, and improved cardiovascular endurance.

- *Mitigating Plateau Phenomenon:* One of the primary goals of metabolic confusion is to avoid the emergence of weight loss plateaus. When a person's body grows used to a certain habit, it develops higher efficiency in energy conservation, which may result in a plateau in development. Individuals may successfully encourage their bodies to continually adapt by changing parameters such as calorie intake and exercise regularly, avoiding performance plateaus, and maintaining an active metabolism.

- *Hormonal Response:* Changes in metabolism may affect the hormonal milieu linked with metabolic processes, such as insulin, leptin, and thyroid hormones. Hormonal oscillations have an important role in regulating appetite, fat storage, and energy expenditure, aiding weight loss and improving body composition.

- *Although the term "metabolic confusion" may look excessive,* this strategy stresses maintaining a healthy and balanced diet as well as participating in frequent exercise. The significance of consistency cannot be emphasized, since the approach to the issue is expressly designed to provide long-term results, preferring long-term sustainability above rapid, fleeting changes.

- *Individual Variability:* It is important to recognize that individual responses to metabolic confusion may differ. Several variables, including genetic predisposition, increasing age, gender, and pre-existing health conditions, may influence the physiological reaction of the body to this specific approach. As a result, before making significant changes to one's food and physical activity routine, it is best to tailor the plan to individual needs and get advice from a healthcare practitioner.

Understanding the Relationship Between Hormones and Metabolic Rate

Hormones of the Thyroid:

Consider your thyroid gland to be the command and control center for your metabolism. It generates the hormones thyroxine (T4) and triiodothyronine (T3) (T3). These hormones function as the gas pedal that controls the speed of your metabolic engine. They have an impact on key activities such as the rate at which your heart beats, your body temperature, and, most significantly, the efficiency with which your cells consume energy. When these hormone levels are low (hypothyroidism), your metabolic engine slows down, which may contribute to weight gain and sluggishness. When these hormone levels are elevated (hyperthyroidism), your metabolic engine speeds up, perhaps resulting in weight reduction and greater energy.

Insulin:

Consider insulin to be the key that allows your cells to consume glucose (sugar) from your bloodstream for energy or storage. It is generated by your pancreas and plays an important role in metabolism. When you eat, your body produces insulin to assist your cells in absorbing glucose. Your cells react less efficiently if you become insulin resistant, which may occur as a result of bad lifestyle practices. This may result in high blood sugar levels and decreased metabolic efficiency.

Leptin:

Consider leptin to be your body's satiety message. It is produced by your fat cells and communicates to your brain that you are full. This hormone acts like a traffic light, signaling, "Stop eating, you're full!" Leptin is essential for managing your body weight and metabolism. When your brain develops resistant to leptin signals, you may feel hungry and find it difficult to maintain a healthy weight.

Ghrelin:

Ghrelin is the hormone that causes your stomach to grumble. Ghrelin is created in the stomach and is your body's way of saying, "Hey, it's time to eat!" Ghrelin levels increase before meals, pushing you to seek food. It's similar to your body's hunger signal. This hormone also affects how your body consumes energy, which affects your metabolic rate.

Cortisol:

Consider cortisol to be your body's stress response. During stressful events, your adrenal glands release it. While it aids in stress management, persistently increased cortisol levels might have negative consequences. Consider cortisol to be a signal that instructs your body to retain fat, particularly around your waist. This may have an impact on how your body utilizes energy and your overall body composition.

Hormone of Growth:

Consider growth hormone (GH) to be your body's repair and restoration team. It is generated by your pituitary gland and is important for muscular development, metabolism, and other functions. GH aids in the breakdown of fats for energy and promotes your body to burn fat for fuel. This directly affects your metabolic rate and how your body utilizes energy.

Estrogen and Testosterone (Sex Hormones):

Consider sexual hormones to be the sculptors of your body's composition. Estrogen in women and testosterone in males influence how your body stores fat, develops muscle and expands. These hormones may impact your metabolic rate and how your body uses energy when they change, such as during menopause or andropause.

Age and Metabolic Rate:

Consider your hormones to be the conductors of a symphony. This symphony alters as you age, and hormonal adjustments occur. Both men and women have a drop in sperm production, which affects muscle mass, fat distribution, and general metabolism. The alterations in this symphony may affect how effectively your metabolic engine functions.

Metabolic Confusion Diet Principles

Macronutrient Cycling

Let us get more into the concept of cycling macronutrients, namely carbohydrates, proteins, and lipids.

Cycling Macronutrients to Improve Nutrition

Consider the human body as a finely tuned device that requires a harmonic blending of many energy sources to work optimally. The fuel source is made up of three major macronutrients: carbohydrates, proteins, and lipids. The concept of macronutrient cycling involves purposely changing the amounts and ratios of these key nutrients in one's food intake over time. This technique offers a plethora of benefits that contribute to one's overall health and fitness goals.

Carbohydrates as the Primary Energy Source

Carbohydrates may be thought of as the primary source of energy that fuels the physiological functions of the human body. They provide the energy required for everyday actions ranging from simple walking to more intense physical effort. Carbohydrates, like quickly combusting logs in a fire, deliver an instant boost of energy. Carbohydrate cycling is the technique of adjusting carbohydrate ingestion based on one's level of physical activity. It may be required to increase carbohydrate intake during times of increased physical activity or participation in severe exercise regimens to replenish depleted glycogen stores and satisfy the higher energy demands put on the body.

Proteins: The Building Blocks of Muscular Development

Proteins are essential components for the repair and maintenance of biological systems. Consider them to be the workers who are engaged in the process of repairing the physical structure that is your corporeal body. The technique of managing protein intake in the context of cycling requires making a conscious effort to get an adequate amount of this crucial nutrient to aid in the process of muscle repair and growth. During times of increased physical activity or strength training, it may be prudent to slightly increase protein intake to supply the required building blocks for muscle recuperation and development.

Fats: Long-Term Energy and Vital Functions

Fats may be thought of as slow-burning logs in a fire, providing a prolonged release of energy over a long period. They are essential in various physiological processes, including hormone production and the digestion of fat-soluble vitamins. The notion of cycling fats entails consuming healthful fat sources in suitable and well-proportioned amounts. Although fats are not the primary source of immediate energy, they are vital for overall health and may be especially beneficial during times of lower-intensity exercise or restorative processes.

The Benefits of Cycling:

- *Improved Performance:* By tailoring one's macronutrient intake to their level of physical activity, people may provide their body with the right amount and quality of energy. This phenomenon can improve workout performance and increase energy levels.

- *Carbohydrate cycling,* or the deliberate modulation of carbohydrate consumption, is a successful technique for both optimizing fat loss and retaining lean muscle composition. Sufficient protein intake aids in the growth and maintenance of muscle tissue, while the inclusion of healthy fats in one's diet aids in the preservation of a harmonious hormonal balance.

- *The capacity of an individual's metabolism* to adapt and modify in response to variations in macronutrient ratios is referred to as metabolic flexibility. Changing these ratios regularly is thought to enhance metabolic plasticity. This condition impairs the body's capacity to optimize the digestion of a certain nutrient, perhaps leading to plateaus.

- *Nutrient optimization:* The method of cycling macronutrients makes it easier to attain a balanced intake of essential nutrients. Every macronutrient has specific benefits, and by including cycling in your diet, you can ensure that your body obtains a diverse spectrum of critical nutrients.

Caloric Variation: The Secret to Avoiding Plateaus

Caloric variety is a strategic strategy for avoiding plateaus experienced in the pursuit of health and fitness goals. It comprises deliberately changing one's daily calorie intake, preventing the body from adapting to a steady caloric routine. This planned calorie variability aids in revitalizing metabolic systems, improving adipose tissue decrease, and enhancing overall results. Let us go into the complexities of caloric variation:

Caloric Variation Deconstructed:

When seen as a flexible organism, it is clear that maintaining a consistent caloric balance throughout time may result in metabolic homeostasis. This balance often results in a plateau—a point at which weight loss or muscle building slows or stops completely. Caloric variation plays a critical function in this situation.

Calorie variation refers to the cyclical modification of one's daily caloric intake. The oscillation between times of high caloric consumption and periods of low caloric consumption serves as a strategy to avoid habituation. The uncertainty of energy supply reduces the proclivity for metabolic adaption.

Enhancing Metabolic Activity: Metabolic activities are analogous to a controlled fire. A constant supply of the same fuel (calories) may cause a slowing similar to fading flames. In contrast, fueling the fire with occasional increments or intensities increases its vitality.

Similarly, caloric variety revs up metabolic processes and prevents complacency.

Overcoming Stagnation: The route to fitness goals, like an adventure with rest stops, necessitates periodic diversions. The caloric variety reflects these halts, ensuring that one's progress does not follow a boring linear pattern.

Individualization and Longevity: Caloric variance occurs as a result of individualization. To accommodate different goals, activity levels, and preferences, the technique must be meticulously calibrated. The goal is neither extreme calorie restriction on low days nor excessive indulgence on high days, but rather a controlled fluctuation that induces a positive adaptive response. The long-term character of this strategy is critical.

Optimizing Lipolysis and Myogenesis: Caloric variation creates a favorable metabolic environment that promotes increased lipid mobilization for energy expenditure. This is the foundation for accelerated adipose tissue decrease. Furthermore, the technique protects muscle preservation and development by providing the necessary energy for intense exercises and the subsequent recuperation phase.

Hormonal Equilibrium: Caloric variety helps to maintain hormonal balance, notably for hormones like leptin and thyroid hormones. These regulatory proteins are critical in modulating metabolic processes and satiety responses. Avoiding prolonged calorie restriction protects against hormonal abnormalities, which might otherwise stymie improvement.

Intermittent Fasting and its Relationship to Metabolic Confusion

Intermittent fasting (IF) and metabolic confusion are two independent but complimentary ways to optimize metabolic health and general well-being. Intermittent fasting includes cycling between eating and fasting phases, while metabolic confusion is caused by variable nutritional and activity characteristics. Understanding their synergy may help explain how these treatments might work together to improve metabolic flexibility and generate beneficial physiological outcomes.

Quick Review on Intermittent Fasting

Intermittent fasting is a kind of eating habit that consists of cycles of eating and not eating. It's similar to scheduling meals and snacks and then giving your body a vacation from eating. This may assist your body in burning stored fat for energy and repairing cells.

A Brief Overview of Metabolic Confusion:

The goal of metabolic confusion is to keep your body guessing. You change things up instead of sticking to the same routine. You consume more calories at times than others. You adjust the meals you consume and your workout regimens. This keeps your body from becoming too comfy, allowing you to burn fat and develop muscle more effectively.

How They Work Together:

Intermittent fasting causes your body to utilize its fat reserves for energy during fasting periods. When you have metabolic confusion, your body becomes even more adept at using those fat reserves. This collaboration allows you to reduce weight more successfully.

Insulin and Hormone Support: Both intermittent fasting and metabolic confusion may improve your body's response to insulin, which is beneficial for blood sugar management. They also collaborate to regulate other hormones that aid in metabolism.

Being Metabolism-Flexible: Consider how your body can switch between utilizing multiple forms of energy, similar to how a vehicle can switch between using gas and electricity. Intermittent fasting teaches your body how to utilize many sorts of energy sources. Metabolic confusion ensures that your body alternates between these sources. This combination aids with weight management.

Avoiding Stuck Points: Our body might get used to the same routine and cease adjusting. This is referred to as reaching a plateau. When you combine intermittent fasting with metabolic confusion, your body continues to change and does not get stagnant. This allows you to continue making progress on your fitness quest.

Intermittent fasting may assist your cells in cleaning up and repairing themselves. When you add metabolic confusion, your cells get various nutrients at different times, which aids in their repair and maintenance.

Important Notes:

Remember that, although these two tactics complement each other nicely, everyone is unique. What works for one individual may not work for another. Before making major changes to your dietary and exercise routines, consult with specialists such as physicians or dietitians.

Intermittent fasting and metabolic confusion work together to disrupt your body's metabolism. They work together to help you burn fat, balance hormones, maintain energy flexibility, prevent plateaus, and even conduct some cellular cleaning. Using these tactics in tandem may provide a significant boost on your way to greater health and fitness.

Creating a Meal Plan for Metabolic Confusion

Designing a Balanced Endomorph Diet: Nutrient Ratios

Creating a nutritionally balanced diet for endomorphs requires careful consideration of nutrient ratios that are compatible with their unique metabolic and physiological features. Given their proclivity for increased fat accumulation, the formulation of food distribution is critical, to facilitate fat loss, preserve lean muscle mass, and foster overall well-being. The following discussion elucidates the key nutritional ratios necessary for developing a sensible diet for endomorphs:

Protein Consumption:

Maintaining Lean Muscle Endomorphs' dietary routine should emphasize the importance of protein intake, which is critical for the maintenance of lean muscle mass while pursuing fat reduction goals. A protein composition of roughly 25-30% of total daily calorie intake serves as a starting point. Lean proteins such as chicken, fish, lean meats, eggs, lentils, and plant-based alternatives are ideal sources.

Carbohydrates: Metabolic Substrates Provision

A sensible carbohydrate allocation of 40-45 percent of daily calorie intake is advised. It is recommended to consume complex carbohydrates, which are mostly sourced from whole grains, fruits, vegetables, and legumes. This option enhances continuous energy supply as well as the incorporation of dietary fiber, which is essential for satiety management and digestive health.

Dietary Fats: Important Lipids for Metabolic Balance

Fats should account for 25-30% of total daily calorie intake. Healthy fats should be obtained mostly from avocados, nuts, seeds, olive oil, and omega-3-rich fatty seafood. These lipid components are essential for hormone synthesis, energy generation, and overall physiological function.

Fiber Promotes Satiety and Metabolic Efficiency

Endomorphs place a premium on the incorporation of dietary fiber. Ample consumption of whole grains, fruits, vegetables, legumes, and nuts offers the necessary fiber content, which aids in satiety, calorie intake management, and digestive process optimization.

Micronutrients: The Building Blocks of Metabolic Homeostasis

Micronutrients, such as vitamins and minerals, play critical roles in metabolic pathways, energy production, and general homeostasis. A diversified array of colored fruits and vegetables should be prioritized to provide a wide range of vital micronutrients. Supplemental interventions should be used sparingly and ideally under expert supervision.

The Hydromineral Nexus in Hydration

Hydration is an important aspect of a healthy diet that is frequently overlooked. Hydration promotes metabolic efficiency, improves digestion, and maintains physiological balance. Adopting sufficient hydration strategies is so critical.

Portion Control: Caloric Balance and Body Composition

Portion control is critical to calorie control, which is a key component of weight management. While nutritional ratios are important, caloric quantity remains a key factor. Mindful portion control and attentive calorie accounting are both effective methods.

Chronobiological Influences on Temporal Nutrient Distribution

The distribution of nutrients across time is critical for metabolic stability. Dispersing meals and snacks throughout the day reduces changes in blood glucose levels, alleviates hunger sensations, and offers long-term energy reserves. Getting enough protein at each meal promotes muscle retention.

Individual Variability: Awareness of Heterogeneity

Individual reactions to specified nutritional ratios are characterized by heterogeneity. Self-monitoring is critical, as is intuitive reactivity to body stimuli. For specialized nutritional structure, it is best to seek the advice of healthcare specialists, especially certified dietitians.

Longitudinal Perspective on Perseverance and Sustained Endeavor

The development of a balanced food routine for endomorphs goes beyond short-term goals. Consistency, patience, and steady advancement are critical for fostering long-term change and solidifying the transition into a sustainable lifestyle paradigm.

7 Days Meal Plans for Various Caloric Intakes

Here are seven-day meal plans for three different caloric intakes: 1500, 2000, and 2500 calories. These meal plans are designed to give a well-balanced approach to nutrition and may be tailored to individual tastes and dietary requirements.

Meal Plan for 1500 Calories

Breakfast on Day 1:

- Scrambled eggs with spinach and tomatoes, whole-grain bread
- Salad with grilled chicken, mixed greens, cucumbers, bell peppers, and balsamic vinaigrette for lunch
- Snack: grapes with Greek yogurt
- Baked salmon, quinoa, and steamed broccoli for dinner

Day 2:

- Oatmeal with sliced banana and almond butter for breakfast
- Lunch: Whole-grain tortilla wrap with turkey and avocado

- Carrot and celery sticks with hummus for a snack

- Stir-fried tofu with mixed veggies and brown rice for dinner

Day 3:

- Greek yogurt parfait with granola and mixed berries for breakfast

- Soup with chickpeas and vegetables for lunch, with a whole-grain roll

- Handful of almonds as a snack

- Dinner will consist of grilled lean steak, baked sweet potatoes, and asparagus.

Day 4:

- Whole-grain pancakes with cottage cheese and sliced strawberries for breakfast

- Quinoa and black bean dish with salsa and avocado for lunch

- Apple slices with peanut butter as a snack

- Baked chicken breast, sautéed zucchini, and quinoa for dinner

Day 5:

- Veggie omelet with whole-grain bread for breakfast

- Lentil salad with mixed greens, feta cheese, and vinaigrette for lunch

- Cottage cheese with pineapple chunks as a snack

- Dinner will consist of grilled salmon, steaming green beans, and wild rice.

Day 6:

- Smoothie with spinach, banana, protein powder, and almond milk for breakfast
- Salad with whole-grain pasta, veggies, and grilled chicken for lunch
- Rice cakes with hummus and cucumber slices as a snack
- Tofu stir-fry with brown rice and snap peas for dinner

Day 7:

- Whole-grain bread with avocado and poached egg for breakfast
- Lunch: Turkey and veggie wrap with salad on the side
- Trail mix with nuts and dried fruits as a snack
- Baked fish, quinoa, and roasted Brussels sprouts for dinner

Meal Plan for 2500 Calories

Day 1:

- Veggie-packed omelet with whole-grain bread and avocado for breakfast
- Snack for mid-morning: Greek yogurt with mixed almonds and honey

- Grilled chicken breast with quinoa, mixed veggies, and an olive oil dressing for lunch
- Snack in the afternoon: Hummus with whole-grain pita and carrot sticks
- Salmon fillet, sweet potato mash, and steamed broccoli for dinner
- Evening Snack: Cottage cheese with fruit and honey drizzle

Day 2

- Breakfast tortilla with scrambled eggs, black beans, cheese, and salsa.
- Snack for mid-morning: apple slices with almond butter
- Salad with turkey and avocado with mixed greens, almonds, seeds, and balsamic vinaigrette for lunch
- Snack during the afternoon: trail mix with dried fruits and mixed nuts
- Dinner will consist of grilled steak, quinoa, roasted veggies, and a side salad.
- Snack in the evening: Greek yogurt with granola and berries

Day 3:

- Whole-grain pancakes with a selection of fresh fruits and maple syrup for breakfast.
- Snack for mid-morning: rice cakes with peanut butter and banana slices

- Brown rice with chickpea and veggie curry for lunch
- Snack in the afternoon: mixed fruit salad with cottage cheese
- Baked chicken thighs, sweet potato wedges, and asparagus for dinner
- Snack for the evening: a handful of mixed nuts

Day 4:

- Smoothie with spinach, banana, berries, protein powder, and almond milk for breakfast
- Snack for mid-morning: Greek yogurt parfait with granola and mixed nuts
- Lunch consists of a grilled veggie and hummus wrap with a side salad.
- Snack during the afternoon: rice cakes with avocado and tomato slices
- Fish tacos with whole-grain tortillas, coleslaw, and salsa for dinner
- Snack in the evening: cheese and whole-grain crackers

Day 5:

- Scrambled eggs with smoked salmon and whole-grain bread for breakfast
- Snack for mid-morning: mixed fruit and cottage cheese
- Quinoa and black bean salad with avocado, mixed greens, and vinaigrette for lunch

- Snack in the afternoon: Nut butter and banana sandwich on whole-grain bread
- Grilled shrimp skewers, brown rice, and grilled veggies for dinner
- Snack for the evening: a handful of trail mix

Day 6:

- Oatmeal with a mix of nuts, seeds, and dried fruits for breakfast
- Snack for mid-morning: Greek yogurt with honey and chopped mixed nuts
- Lunch: Caesar salad with grilled chicken and whole-grain croutons
- Snack during the afternoon: Apple slices with cheese
- Dinner consists of turkey meatballs, whole-grain pasta, marinara sauce, and steamed greens.
- Snack for the evening: rice cakes with hummus and cucumber slices

Day 7:

- Breakfast tortilla with scrambled eggs, veggies, cheese, and salsa.
- Snack for mid-morning: cottage cheese with mixed berries and honey drizzle

- Tuna salad with mixed greens, olives, cherry tomatoes, and an olive oil dressing for lunch
- Snack in the afternoon: whole-grain crackers with guacamole
- Stir-fried tofu with veggies, brown rice, and teriyaki sauce for dinner
- Evening Snack: Greek yogurt with chopped almonds and cinnamon sprinkled on top

Meal Plan for 2000 Calories

Day 1:

- Scrambled eggs with sautéed spinach and whole-grain bread for breakfast
- Lunch salad with grilled chicken, mixed greens, cherry tomatoes, cucumbers, and vinaigrette
- Greek yogurt with a handful of mixed berries as a snack
- Baked salmon with quinoa and roasted asparagus for dinner

Day 2:

- Breakfast: Whole-grain oatmeal with sliced bananas, chopped almonds, and honey drizzle
- Lunch: Turkey and avocado wrap with whole-grain tortilla and salad on the side
- Carrot and celery sticks with hummus for a snack

- Stir-fried tofu with broccoli, bell peppers, and brown rice for dinner

Day 3:

- Greek yogurt parfait with oats and other fruits for breakfast
- Lentil and vegetable soup with whole-grain bread for lunch
- Handful of almonds as a snack
- Grilled chicken breast with sweet potato mash and steamed green beans for dinner

Day 4:

- Smoothie with mixed berries, spinach, protein powder, and almond milk for breakfast
- Salad of chickpeas and quinoa with mixed veggies and a lemon-tahini dressing for lunch
- Apple slices with almond butter as a snack
- Baked fish with roasted veggies and wild rice for dinner

Day 5:

- Whole-grain bread with avocado and a poached egg for breakfast
- Lunch: Stir-fried turkey and vegetables with brown rice
- Cottage cheese with pineapple chunks as a snack
- Dinner is grilled lean steak with quinoa and steamed broccoli.

Day 6:

- Veggie omelet with feta cheese and whole-grain bread for breakfast
- Lunch: Hummus and grilled veggie wrap with mixed greens on the side
- Snack: a combination of nuts and dry fruits
- Baked chicken thighs with quinoa and sautéed spinach for dinner

Day 7:

- Whole-grain pancakes with mixed berries and a dab of Greek yogurt for breakfast
- Quinoa and black bean dish with avocado, salsa, and a side salad for lunch
- Rice cakes with peanut butter as a snack
- Dinner: grilled fish with roasted sweet potatoes and Brussels sprouts on the side

Meal Frequency and Timing for Best Results

Meal frequency and timing are critical elements in optimizing nutrition and achieving your health and fitness goals. Tailoring your food habits to your needs and goals may help with energy balance, metabolic support, and overall well-being. The following is a breakdown of optimum meal time and frequency:

Understanding the Importance of Meal Frequency and Timing

The time and frequency of our meals are critical parts of our eating habits that have a significant influence on our metabolic and physiological processes. Meal planning throughout the day can alter energy levels, metabolic efficiency, and general well-being. Investigating the complexities of meal time and frequency may bring useful insights on how to use these elements to our benefit.

Igniting the Metabolic Furnace for Breakfast

Starting the day with a well-balanced breakfast has emerged as a critical discipline. Breakfast is the figurative spark that ignites our metabolic furnace, stimulating energy generation and kicking off the chain reaction of biochemical events that support physiological activity. A breakfast high in protein, complex carbs, and healthy fats lays the groundwork for long-term energy release.

Mid-Morning Snack: Keeping Energy Balance

A mid-morning snack presents itself as a smart move, especially if the time between breakfast and lunch is long. This interlude maintains energy homeostasis while mitigating possible energy lulls. Choosing a snack high in protein and fiber promotes satiety and acts as a nutritional bridge until the next meal.

Lunch: Nutrient Resupply and Sustenance

Lunch serves as a critical break, allowing for the replenishment of nutrients and the maintenance of physiological equilibrium. A well-balanced meal consists of a combination of lean proteins, complex carbs, and healthy fats. This formula produces a burst of prolonged energy, bolstering cognitive performance and physical stamina.

Snack for the Afternoon: Reducing Afternoon Fatigue

As the afternoon passes, including an afternoon snack might help to avoid weariness and excessive hunger, which can lead to overindulgence at dinner. Choosing a snack that has both protein and fiber promotes satiety while avoiding abrupt blood sugar changes.

Dinner: Nourishment Culmination

Dinner is the conclusion of daily sustenance, requiring a careful orchestration of nutrients to satisfy both physiological needs and sensory delight. Dinner, like lunch, should include lean meats, complex carbs, and plenty of veggies. Allowing for a short period between meals and sleep promotes good digestion and sleep quality.

Evening Snack (Optional): Make Mindful Decisions

If the need arises, an evening snack might be a wise choice if it adheres to the principles of portion control and nutritional density. Satiety and nutritional prudence may be found in foods like cottage cheese with fruit or a little serving of whole-grain cereal.

A Customized Approach to Meal Frequency

The frequency of meals and snacks needs personalized calibration. This customization is guided by preferences, activity levels, and personal circadian cycles. This may vary from a three-meal paradigm to a more elaborate pattern that includes five to six smaller meals and snacks. The goal is to develop a routine that ideally supports energy levels while also aligning with one's lifestyle.

Holistic Hydration: A Fundamental Basis

Beyond food, the subject of hydration takes center stage. Consistent water consumption throughout the day is critical for metabolic vigor, nutritional transport, and physiological balance. The periodicity of feeding is supplemented by enough hydration.

A Contemplative Approach to Mindful Eating

The habit of mindful eating emerges as a vital companion amid the orchestration of meal time and frequency. Consciously attention to hunger indicators, relishing each mouthful, and building an attuned connection with our bodies' signals all contribute to a satisfying eating experience.

Using Metabolic Confusion Workouts

Diet and Exercise: Why Both Are Important

Consider nutrition and exercise to be two dancing partners on a health journey, moving in unison to produce a dazzling well-being choreography. These disparate components have a deep bond that transcends ordinary cohabitation. Let us delve into why this dynamic combination is so important, revealing its linked importance.

Weight Management Dynamic Duo

- Consider food and exercise to be the perfect weight-management tag team. A well-balanced diet helps to control calorie intake, while activity burns those calories, resulting in a healthy calorie balance. This teamwork becomes a powerful weight loss or weight maintenance method.

Muscle Sculpting Through Collaboration

- When it comes to muscles, diet, and exercise dance in a fascinating tango. Protein in your diet acts as the building blocks for muscle repair and development. Exercise, particularly strength training, then stimulates muscle fibers to adapt and thrive.

Metabolism: An Efficient Symphony

- Diet and exercise work together to create a metabolic symphony. A well-balanced diet supports metabolic processes by making nutrients easily accessible for energy generation. Simultaneously, regular exercise raises metabolic rate, maximizing energy usage and allowing fat reserves to be used as fuel.

Harmony and Hormones

- Consider nutrition and exercise to be the masters of hormone balance. A diet high in nutrients such as healthy fats and complex carbohydrates promotes hormone synthesis. Meanwhile, exercise releases endorphins and other mood-enhancing chemicals, improving emotional balance.

Heart Health: A Pairing

- Diet and exercise work in unison to improve cardiovascular health. A heart-healthy diet rich in fiber, antioxidants, and omega-3 fatty acids lowers blood pressure and cholesterol. Simultaneously, exercise improves the function of the heart, improving circulation and protecting against heart disease.

Mental Agility: A Clarity Choreography

- The interaction of nutrition and exercise has a greater impact on mental agility. Nutrient-dense meals supply the building blocks for the brain, while physical exercise increases cerebral blood flow, increasing cognitive ability.

Lifetime Vibration

- Diet and exercise together form an elixir for lifespan and illness prevention. A nutritious diet combined with regular exercise functions as a barrier against chronic diseases, allowing people to enjoy bright health throughout their lives.

Serenade to Happiness

- This synergistic dance tugs at the psychological well-being strings. A healthy diet promotes neurotransmitter production, which influences mood. Physical exercise, particularly mindful activities, develops as a stress-relieving pattern that fosters mental resilience.

Goal-oriented Choreography

- Recognizing the relationship between nutrition and exercise involves tailoring your routine to your goals. You may modify your food choices and exercise regimens to meet particular objectives, such as losing weight, increasing muscle, or simply embracing overall vigor.

Workout Plans for Endomorph Women

Creating workout programs that are suited to the particular qualities of endomorph women demands a thorough study of their physiological characteristics. Endomorphs often have a larger percentage of body fat and a slower metabolic rate. Nonetheless, their unique constitution does not stop them from reaching fitness goals; rather, it emphasizes the need to create tailored training routines that are in sync with their body composition. Let's have a look at the sophisticated process of developing training programs that are tailored to the unique demands of endomorph women:

- **Interval Cardiovascular Exercise:** Interval cardio workouts have emerged as an important component for caloric expenditure and cardiovascular health. Interval training was developed as a strategic option for endomorph women. This method incorporates short bursts of high-intensity training, such as sprints or plyometric movements, followed by short bursts of low-intensity recuperation. Endomorphs may improve calorie burn, boost metabolism, and avoid adaption by adopting this technique.

- **Strength training is emphasized:** Strength training is essential for increasing metabolic rate and improving body shape. Prioritize complex activities such as squats, deadlifts, and lunges, which engage many muscular groups at the same time. Endomorph women may promote muscular development and metabolic efficiency by aiming for moderate to significant resistance levels while gradually increasing the load.

- **Utilizing Resistance Training:** Using resistance bands or bodyweight workouts may help you build lean muscular mass. This becomes useful in increasing metabolic activity and promoting fat reduction, which is an important factor for endomorphs seeking ideal body composition.

- **Making Use of High-Intensity Interval Training (HIIT):** HIIT exercises are appealing to endomorph women because of their extraordinary ability to boost metabolism and fat burning. HIIT boosts the body's physiological reactions by alternating short bursts of strenuous activity with short rest periods, driving calorie expenditure, and post-exercise effects.

- **Accept Circuit Training:** Circuit training, which combines aerobic and strength-based workouts in fast succession, provides a complete workout regimen. This method increases calorie burn, improves muscular endurance, and promotes cardiovascular fitness, making it an excellent alternative for endomorphs seeking fat reduction and muscle refinement.

- **Developing Flexibility and Mobility:** Prioritizing flexibility and mobility therapies, such as yoga or Pilates, helps overall well-being. These methods improve joint flexibility, reduce tension, and speed up post-workout recovery, making them an important part of the program.

- **Reflecting on Rest and Recovery:** Endomorph women should prioritize rest days to avoid overtraining and enhance muscle recovery. A healthy training regimen is fostered by prioritizing appropriate sleep, good food choices, and active recovery strategies such as foam rolling.

- **Nutritional Planning:** Because endomorphs are inclined to weight gain, a rigorous nutritional strategy is required. Make a nutrient-dense diet a priority, including whole foods, lean protein sources, healthy fats, and complex carbs. Portion management is critical, and meals should be tailored to your energy expenditure and fitness goals.

- **The Importance of Consistency:** Sustained consistency is the key to reaching fitness objectives. Endomorph women must commit to regular workout sessions and a well-balanced food regimen over time to see long-term results.

- **Recruit Professional Help:** Working with a skilled fitness expert or a licensed nutritionist who understands the subtleties of endomorph body types is a wise move. These professionals can help you design a personalized workout and nutrition plan that fits your goals, limits, and preferences.

Overcoming Obstacles and Maintaining Consistency

Managing Cravings and Emotional Eating

The complex terrain of cravings and emotional eating is frequent, yet it is controllable with the correct thoughts and tactics. These inclinations may occasionally lead us astray from our dietary objectives, but you can reclaim control of your eating habits by diving into the dynamics at work and using effective ways. Here's a detailed approach to navigating cravings and emotional eating with grace:

- **Decipher Trigger Points:** Begin by identifying the triggers that cause your cravings and emotional eating bouts. These triggers might include tension, boredom, melancholy, or the surroundings in which you find yourself. By identifying these triggers, you can control them ahead of time.

- **Distinguish between Hunger and Desires:** Recognize the differences between actual bodily hunger and emotional cravings. When the need to eat occurs, stop and consider if your body genuinely requires nourishment or whether it is an emotional response. This knowledge is a potent strategy for reducing emotional eating.

- **Mindful Eating:** Incorporate awareness into your eating regimen. This entails thoroughly immersing oneself in the sensory experience of your meals. Engage your senses, take each mouthful slowly, and enjoy the textures and tastes. This exercise strengthens your connection to your body's hunger and fullness signals.

- **Holistic Emotional Coping:** Instead of using food as an emotional shelter, look into other options for dealing with emotions. Engage in things that you like, such as jogging, meditating, drawing, or just relaxing with a book. These options provide productive channels for emotional release.

- **Balanced Meals:** Create a culinary plan that promotes balance. Make sure your meals include a variety of nutrients, including protein, healthy fats, and complex carbs. This dietary balance regulates blood sugar levels, reducing extreme cravings.

- **Out of Sight, Out of Mind:** Keep trigger foods out of sight to reduce temptation. Choose healthier options that are easily available, favorably influencing your decisions.

- **Hydration, the Unseen Friend:** Dehydration sometimes masquerades as hunger or urges. Maintain your hydration levels throughout the day by drinking plenty of water, which reduces the probability of unnecessary eating.

- **Portion Control:** If you must indulge in a desire, do it carefully and in moderation. Portion management is an excellent ally in the fight to manage desires without deviating from your objectives.

- **Anticipatory Snacking:** Before entering settings that may induce desires, have a nutritious snack. This preventative technique prevents insatiable hunger and rash decisions.

- **Create a Support System:** Tell someone about your experience, whether it's a friend, family member, or a counselor. During difficult times, a support system provides encouragement, accountability, and a cushion.

- **Keep a Food Diary:** Write down your eating habits, feelings, and triggers in a diary. This introspective activity reveals trends and equips you with the knowledge to make educated choices about emotional eating.

- **Cultivate Self-Compassion:** Accept self-kindness and accept that mistakes are a part of the process. Instead of dwelling on your missteps, consider the forward-thinking decisions you may make in the future.

Dining Out and Navigating Social Situations

Starting a better eating path does not have to mean giving up social activities or dining experiences. With a rigorous approach and careful preparation, you may enjoy social gatherings while still achieving your health goals. Here's a helpful tip on negotiating social settings while eating out:

- **Menu Evaluation in Advance:** Before going out to eat, be proactive and go over the menu online, if available. This proactive technique allows you to make educated judgments ahead of time, reducing impulsive decisions at the table.

- **Prudent Location Selection:** Choose restaurants with a wide variety of nutritional selections on their menu. This broadens your options and promotes health-conscious choices without feeling restricted.

- **Ordering with Conscience:** When making your order, choose grilling, baking, or steaming over fried or strongly sautéed options. Dressings and sauces should be offered on the side, giving you discretion over portion size.

- **Portion Control:** It should be noted that restaurant serving sizes often surpass standard standards. Consider sharing an entrée with a buddy, ordering a lesser quantity, or saving half of your meal for another time.

- **Accept Vegetable Abundance:** Choose recipes that are high in veggies, healthful grains, and lean protein sources. These nutrient-dense options satisfy hunger while also providing critical nutrients.

- **Beverage Administration:** Favor water, unsweetened tea, or sparkling water to up your beverage game. Limit your intake of sugary drinks and alcohol, which may provide extra calories with no nutritious benefit.

- **Preparation for Social Interaction:** Prioritize discussion and social engagement before beginning your meal. This methodical technique helps your body to detect genuine hunger signals, preventing overindulgence caused by distractions.

- **Gastronomy with Awareness:** Begin practicing mindful eating, which includes enjoying each piece, chewing slowly, and sometimes setting utensils aside. This promotes a stronger relationship with your food, preventing hastiness.

- **Indulgence with Purpose:** If a delicacy or dessert calls, enjoy with intention and mindfulness. Immerse yourself in the experience, savoring each mouthful and paying attention to your body's reactions.

- **Special Occasions Stratagem:** For major occasions, plan ahead of time by limiting your consumption throughout the day. Choose lighter cuisine before and after the occasion to allow for enjoyment while maintaining balance.

- **Assertively communicate:** Don't be afraid to express your food choices or needs to your companions or the waiter. Many eating locations allow for personalization.

- **Develop Mindful Social Activities:** Develop social efforts that go beyond the world of food. Suggest hikes, museum trips, or other fascinating events that build contact without a culinary emphasis.

- **Center Shift:** Shift the focus away from the food and onto the stimulating fellowship and talk. Conversations and genuine friendships might reduce the food to a secondary position.

- **Accept the Adaptive Mindset:** Remember that periodic indulgence is not only permitted but also beneficial to your overall health. Approach these circumstances with an eye toward improvement rather than an unrealistic goal of perfection.

- **Positive Point of View:** Positively frame your eating out experiences. Consider them chances to practice mindfulness and make decisions that are in line with your overall well-being.

Beyond the Scale: Progress Monitoring

When going on a path to enhance health and fitness, it is critical to understand that progress cannot be evaluated only by numbers on a scale. While weight is an obvious indicator, a full examination considers a variety of factors. Here's an outline of how to measure progress beyond the scale, including both physical and non-physical aspects:

- Body Measurements: Taking measurements of major body parts such as the waist, hips, chest, and limbs regularly offers insight into changes in body composition. Even if weight stays consistent, reductions in measures may indicate changes in fat and muscle proportions.

- Body Composition Analysis: Techniques such as bioelectrical impedance or DEXA scans provide information on body fat and lean muscle mass. This information offers a more accurate picture of how your body's composition varies.

- Fitness Levels: It is critical to track your fitness progress. Running longer distances, lifting heavier weights, or completing more advanced yoga positions may all indicate improved strength, endurance, and flexibility.

- Increased energy levels and less weariness in everyday activities are signs of increased fitness and general well-being.

- Mood and Mental Well-Being: Positive mood swings, lower stress levels, and increased mental clarity are important indicators of improvement. Regular exercise has been shown to improve mental wellness.

- Sleep Quality: Improvements in sleep patterns, such as falling asleep more quickly, having fewer interruptions, and waking up feeling revitalized, indicate favorable changes.

- Clothing Fit: Changes in how your clothing fits or the need to go down a size suggest adjustments in body composition, even if the scale doesn't show any significant changes.

- Track improvements in performance, such as quicker racing times, better endurance, or refined athletic abilities, if you participate in sports endeavors.

- Health Risk Factors: Regular exercise and a well-balanced diet help to improve health indicators such as blood pressure, cholesterol levels, and blood sugar management.

- Digestive Health: Dietary modifications and greater physical activity may be connected to improved digestion, less bloating, and general gut health.

- Self-esteem and body confidence are typically boosted when you see success and good improvements in your life.

- Consistency and Behaviors: Maintaining a regular workout regimen and adhering to healthy habits is a huge achievement. Consistency is essential for obtaining long-term outcomes.

- Shifts to healthy living behaviors, such as cooking more at home, choosing nutrient-rich meals, and practicing mindful eating, suggest a good shift.

- Functional fitness is defined as the capacity to do daily chores with increased ease, such as moving groceries, mounting stairs, or participating in physical activities.

- Building a network of support and accountability, whether via friends. family, or fitness groups, helps to create an atmosphere favorable to success.

Successful Meal Preparation and Recipes

The Importance of Meal Preparation in Long-Term Success

Food planning is a deliberate and proactive approach to meal management that is critical to ensuring long-term success on your road to health and fitness. By devoting time ahead of time to plan, prepare, and arrange your meals, you unleash a slew of advantages that add significantly to your long-term well-being and fitness goals. Here's an instructive summary of the significance of meal planning in long-term success:

- **Nutritional Intake Consistency:** Meal preparing enables you to regularly align with balanced nutrition. The process of precisely organizing your meals helps you make intelligent food choices, reducing the inclination to choose less healthful alternatives impulsively.

- **Mastering Portion Management:** Portion control is at the core of healthy eating. Meal preparation makes this practice easier by allowing you to correctly measure and divide your meals, reducing overeating. This thoughtful approach promotes knowledge of proper portion proportions and assists with calorie control.

- **Time Management Efficiency and Convenience:** In today's fast-paced world, finding time for everyday cooking might be difficult. Meal planning overcomes this difficulty by putting the cooking effort first. It gives you the luxury of leisure during hectic days since your meals are made ahead of time and ready for you.

- **Taming Impulse Decisions:** Hunger and time restrictions sometimes lead to rash, poor dietary choices. By planning your meals, you create a repertory of better choices that are immediately accessible, reducing the temptation to choose less nutritious options.

- **Financial prudence:** Eating out often might put a burden on your wallet. Meal planning enables you to take advantage of the economics of bulk purchasing, resulting in long-term savings. Furthermore, the cost of prepared meals is sometimes less expensive than restaurant expenses.

- **Ingredient Control:** Meal preparation puts you in charge of ingredient choices. This freedom allows you to choose fresh, high-quality ingredients, control flavor, and portion amounts, and avoid unnecessary sweets, harmful fats, and additives.

- **Maintaining Dietary Consistency:** Whether you follow a certain dietary regimen or seek precise macronutrient ratios, meal preparation becomes a vital ally in maintaining persistent consistency. Adherence rises when your meals are consistent with your dietary goals.

- **Liberation from Decision Fatigue:** The everyday variety of food-related options may put a load on the brain. Meal planning relieves the strain of impulsive decision-making, freeing up brain space for other cognitive tasks.

- **Catering to Special Dietary Needs:** Meal planning allows for personalization for persons with dietary restrictions, allergies, or specific health goals. You may meet precise requirements without compromising taste or diversity.

- **Individuals who are engrossed in arduous activities find refuge in meal preparation.** It guarantees that nutritionally balanced meals are always available, even during busy periods when traditional cooking is impossible.

- **Mindful Eating:** With pre-prepared meals, you're ready to participate in mindful consumption. This technique helps you to appreciate each mouthful, building a deeper connection with your food and encouraging healthy digestion.

- **Reduce Food Waste:** Meal planning increases resourcefulness and reduces food waste. Ingredients are used wisely, and leftovers may be recycled for future meals.

Recipes that are both quick and nutrient-dense

1. Greek Yogurt Parfait:

Ingredients:

- 1 cup plain Greek yogurt (low-fat or non-fat)
- 1/2 cup berries, mixed (blueberries, strawberries, raspberries)
- 1 tbsp honey (or maple syrup)
- 2 granola tablespoons

Instructions:

- Layer Greek yogurt, mixed berries, and granola in a glass or dish.
- Drizzle with honey or maple syrup.
- Enjoy your protein-rich, creamy parfait!

Nutritional Information (approximate):

- Calories: 242
- Protein: 17g
- Carbohydrates: 43g
- Fiber: 6g
- Fat: 5g

2. **Oatmeal with Nut Butter and Banana:**

Ingredients:

- Half a cup of rolled oats
- one cup of milk (dairy or plant-based)
- One spoonful of almond butter (peanut, almond, etc.)
- Half a banana, cut
- One-tsp chia seeds (optional)
- For taste, add some cinnamon.

Instructions:

- Follow the directions on the box to cook the oats in milk.
- Add nut butter, sliced bananas, chia seeds, and a dash of cinnamon on top.

Nutritional Information (approximate):

- Calories: 370
- Protein: 14g
- Carbohydrates: 53g
- Fiber: 9g
- Fat: 17g

3. Avocado Toast with Egg:

Ingredients:

- 1 slice whole-grain bread, toasted, 1/2 avocado, mashed

- 1 egg, cooked (fried, scrambled, or poached), add Salt and pepper to taste
- Optional toppings: red pepper flakes, chopped herbs

Instructions:

- Toast the bread and spread it with mashed avocado.
- Serve with a fried egg on top.
- Season with salt, pepper, and any other seasonings you desire.

Nutritional Information (approximate):

- Calories: 310
- Protein: 12g
- Carbohydrates: 19g
- Fiber: 9g
- Fat: 19g

4. Veggie and Cheese Omelette:

Ingredients:

- two eggs
- 1/4 cup of bell peppers, chopped
- one-fourth cup of chopped tomatoes
- 1/4 cup of finely chopped spinach
- 1/4 cup of cheese, shredded (cheddar, mozzarella, etc.)
- Season with salt, pepper, and herbs.

Instructions:

- Whisk eggs in a mixing basin and season with salt and pepper.
- Sauté bell peppers, tomatoes, and spinach in a nonstick skillet until softened.
- Cook until the eggs are set, then pour them over the vegetables.
- Sprinkle shredded cheese on one side of the omelet, fold it in half, and cook until the cheese melts.

Nutritional Information (approximate):

- Calories: 282
- Protein: 23g
- Carbohydrates: 8g
- Fiber: 3g
- Fat: 17g

5. Smoothie Bowl:

Ingredients:

- One banana, frozen
- Half a cup of frozen mixed berries
- half a cup of kale or spinach
- Half a cup of milk (dairy or plant-based)
- One spoonful of almond butter
- Add-ons: cereal, chopped fruit, almonds, and seeds

Instructions:

- Smoothly blend frozen banana, mixed berries, kale or spinach, milk, and nut butter.
- Transfer the blended drink to a bowl.
- Add granola, chopped nuts, seeds, and sliced fruits on top.

Nutritional Information (approximate):

- Calories: 352
- Protein: 12g
- Carbohydrates: 50g
- Fiber: 10g
- Fat: 14g

6. Quinoa Salad with Chickpeas and Veggies:

Ingredients:

- One cup of cooked quinoa
- One cup of rinsed and drained canned chickpeas
- one cup of cucumbers, chopped
- Diced bell peppers, one cup
- 1/4 cup of freshly chopped parsley
- Two tsp of feta cheese (optional)
- Two tsp olive oil
- One lemon's juice
- To taste, add salt and pepper.

Instructions:

- Toss cooked quinoa, chickpeas, cucumber, bell peppers, and parsley in a big bowl.
- Mix the olive oil, lemon juice, salt, and pepper in a small bowl.
- After adding the dressing, thoroughly toss the quinoa mixture.
- If preferred, top with feta cheese sprinkled atop.

Nutritional Information (approximate):

- Calories: 402
- Protein: 13g
- Carbohydrates: 52g
- Fiber: 11g
- Fat: 17g

7. Grilled Chicken Wrap with Hummus and Veggies:

Ingredients:

- One tortilla or wrap made entirely of whole wheat
- 4 ounces of grilled, sliced chicken breast
- Two tsp of hummus
- Half a cup of sliced tomatoes
- Half a cup of cucumbers, sliced
- One-fourth cup of finely chopped lettuce

- To taste, add salt and pepper.

Instructions:

- Spread the hummus evenly over the flattened wrap.
- Top with shredded lettuce, tomatoes, cucumbers, and sliced grilled chicken.
- Add pepper and salt for seasoning.
- Enjoy the wrap after carefully rolling it up.

Nutritional Information (approximate):

- Calories: 351
- Protein: 32g
- Carbohydrates: 25g
- Fiber: 6g
- Fat: 12g

8. Lentil and Vegetable Stir-Fry:

Ingredients:

- one cup of brown or green lentils, cooked
- One cup of assorted stir-fried veggies (broccoli, carrots, bell peppers)
- One tablespoon of olive oil
- Two tsp of soy sauce (low sodium)
- one minced garlic clove
- one tsp finely chopped ginger

- Red pepper flakes crushed (optional)
- Sunflower seeds as a garnish

Instructions:

- Warm up some olive oil in a pan over medium heat.
- Add the grated ginger and minced garlic, and cook for one minute.
- Vegetables should be stir-fried and cooked until just soft.
- Add the soy sauce and cooked lentils and stir. If desired, add some red pepper flakes.
- Cook for a few more minutes to ensure it is well-heated.
- Garnish with sesame seeds before serving.

Nutritional Information (approximate):

- Calories: 352
- Protein: 22g
- Carbohydrates: 53g
- Fiber: 16g
- Fat: 9g

9. Spinach and Chickpea Salad with Tuna:

Ingredients:

- two cups of baby spinach
- 1/2 cup washed and drained canned chickpeas
- One can of drained tuna

- 1/4 cup of red onion, chopped

- 1/4 cup of cucumbers, chopped

- Double-thumb spread balsamic vinaigrette

- To taste, add salt and pepper.

Instructions:

- Baby spinach, chickpeas, tuna, red onion, and cucumber should all be combined in a big dish.

- Over the salad, drizzle the balsamic vinaigrette.

- Add pepper and salt for seasoning.

- Mix well and enjoy your crisp salad.

Nutritional Information (approximate):

- Calories: 306

- Protein: 34g

- Carbohydrates: 21g

- Fiber: 5g

- Fat: 12g

10. Vegetable and Quinoa Stir-Fry:

Ingredients:

- One cup of cooked quinoa

- One cup of assorted stir-fried veggies (zucchini, carrots, snap peas)

- One tablespoon of sesame oil

- Two tsp of soy sauce (low sodium)
- One-tsp rice vinegar
- One tsp honey
- half a tsp finely grated ginger
- Sunflower seeds as a garnish

Instructions:

- Heat the sesame oil in a pan over medium heat.
- Vegetables should be added and sautéed until crisp-tender.
- Combine the soy sauce, rice vinegar, honey, and grated ginger in a small bowl.
- Place the cooked quinoa in the skillet with the veggies and cover with the sauce.
- Stir-fry for a few minutes until well mixed.
- Garnish with sesame seeds before serving.

Nutritional Information (approximate):

- Calories: 356
- Protein: 19g
- Carbohydrates: 53g
- Fiber: 9g
- Fat: 11g

11. Baked Salmon with Roasted Vegetables:

Ingredients:

- 1 salmon fillet (6 oz)
- 1 cup mixed veggies (broccoli, carrots, bell peppers)
- 1 tablespoon olive oil
- Seasonings: salt, pepper, and herbs

Instructions:

- Set oven temperature to 400°F, or 200°C.
- Salmon should be placed on a baking pan and drizzled with lemon juice, zest, and olive oil.
- Add herbs, salt, and pepper for seasoning.
- Arrange a mixture of veggies around the fish.
- Bake the salmon for 15 to 20 minutes, or until it is cooked through, and flakes readily when tested with a fork.

Nutritional Information (approximate):

- Calories: 402
- Protein: 31g
- Carbohydrates: 13g
- Fiber: 4g
- Fat: 27g

12. Chickpea and Vegetable Stir-Fry with Brown Rice:

Ingredients:

- One cup of brown rice, cooked
- One cup of rinsed and drained canned chickpeas
- One cup of assorted stir-fried veggies, such as bell peppers, carrots, and snow peas
- Two tsp of soy sauce (low sodium)
- One tablespoon of sesame oil
- one tsp finely chopped garlic
- optional crushed red pepper flakes

Instructions:

- In a pan over medium heat, warm the sesame oil.
- Stir-fry the veggies after adding the minced garlic. Cook until softened.
- To the pan, add the cooked brown rice and chickpeas.
- If desired, top the mixture with red pepper flakes and soy sauce.
- Stir-fry for a few minutes, or until well hot and completely blended.

Nutritional Information (approximate):

- Calories: 452
- Protein: 15g
- Carbohydrates: 73g

- Fiber: 11g

- Fat: 13g

13. Grilled Chicken with Quinoa and Steamed Broccoli:

Ingredients:

- grilled chicken breast, 4 ounces

- Half a cup of cooked quinoa

- One cup of steaming broccoli

- One tablespoon of olive oil

- Juice from lemons

- Season with salt, pepper, and herbs.

Instructions:

- Lemon juice, olive oil, salt, pepper, and herbs are used to season grilled chicken.

- Accompany the grilled chicken with steamed broccoli and cooked quinoa.

Nutritional Information (approximate):

- Calories: 402

- Protein: 33g

- Carbohydrates: 32g

- Fiber: 8g

- Fat: 16g

14. Lentil and Spinach Salad with Feta:

Ingredients:

- One cup of cooked green lentils
- two cups of baby spinach
- 1/4 cup of feta cheese, crumbled
- 1/4 cup of red onion, chopped
- 1/4 cup of cucumbers, chopped
- 2 tbsp of balsamic vinaigrette
- To taste, add salt and pepper.

Instructions:

- Cooked lentils, baby spinach, feta cheese, red onion, and cucumber should all be combined in a big dish.
- Over the salad, drizzle the balsamic vinaigrette.
- Add pepper and salt for seasoning.
- Once fully combined, enjoy your nutrient-dense salad.

Nutritional Information (approximate):

- Calories: 330
- Protein: 19g
- Carbohydrates: 44g
- Fiber: 12g
- Fat: 11g

15. Veggie and Tofu Stir-Fry with Noodles:

Ingredients:

- One cup of cooked rice or whole wheat noodles
- 4 ounces diced firm tofu
- One cup of assorted stir-fried veggies, such as bell peppers, carrots, and bok choy
- Two tsp of soy sauce (low sodium)
- One tsp of hoisin sauce
- One tsp of sesame oil
- one tsp finely chopped ginger
- chopped green onions for the garnish

Instructions:

- Heat the sesame oil in a pan over medium heat.
- Stir-fry the cubed tofu until it becomes golden brown.
- Add mixed veggies and minced ginger. Sauté the veggies until they are soft.
- Stir in cooked noodles, soy sauce, and hoisin sauce.
- Cook for a few minutes, or until well heated.
- Before serving, sprinkle some chopped green onions on top.

Nutritional Information (approximate):

- Calories: 408
- Protein: 17g

- Carbohydrates: 56g

- Fiber: 9g

- Fat: 12g

16. Greek Yogurt Parfait with Berries and Nuts:

Ingredients:

- 1/2 cup fat-free or low-fat Greek yogurt

- 1/4 cup of berry mixture (strawberries, raspberries, and blueberries)

- 1 tablespoon of finely chopped nuts (walnuts, almonds)

- One tsp honey or maple syrup

Instructions:

- Arrange Greek yogurt, chopped almonds, and mixed berries in a glass or dish.

- Overtop, drizzle some maple syrup or honey.

- Savor your delicious, creamy, protein-packed parfait!

Nutritional Information (approximate):

- Calories: 202

- Protein: 16g

- Carbohydrates: 25g

- Fiber: 5g

- Fat: 6g

17. Dark Chocolate-Dipped Strawberries:

Ingredients:

- Six new strawberries
- Two ounces of dark chocolate (at least 70% cocoa)

Instructions:

- In a microwave-safe dish, melt dark chocolate for 20 seconds at a time, stirring in between.
- Each strawberry should be dipped halfway into the molten chocolate.
- After dipping the strawberries, place them on a dish lined with paper and refrigerate to let the chocolate solidify.
- Savor this tasty, high-antioxidant delight!

Nutritional Information (approximate):

- Calories: 152
- Protein: 4g
- Carbohydrates: 19g
- Fiber: 5g
- Fat: 8g

18. Frozen Banana Bites:

Ingredients:

- One ripe banana, cut.

- Two tsp of nut butter (peanut, almond)
- Two tsp dark chocolate chips

Instructions:

- On one side of the banana slices, spread nut butter.
- Place nut butter in the center of two banana slices and sandwich them together.
- Melt the dark chocolate and dip each banana sandwich into it.
- Transfer to a parchment paper-lined dish and refrigerate until the chocolate solidifies.
- Savor this creamy, frozen treat!

Nutritional Information (approximate):

- Calories: 230
- Protein: 5g
- Carbohydrates: 33g
- Fiber: 5g
- Fat: 10g

19. Chia Seed Pudding with Mixed Berries:

Ingredients:

- Two tsp of chia seeds
- 1/2 cup almond milk, unsweetened (or any milk of choice)
- Half a teaspoon of extract from vanilla

- 1/4 cup of berry mixture (blueberries, raspberries)

Instructions:

- Combine chia seeds, almond milk, and vanilla essence in a dish.
- To make it thicker, give it a good stir and refrigerate for at least two hours or overnight.
- Top with mixed berries before serving.
- Savor your omega-3-rich, high-fiber dessert!

Nutritional Information (approximate):

- Calories: 155
- Protein: 7g
- Carbohydrates: 18g
- Fiber: 12g
- Fat: 9g

20. Baked Apple with Cinnamon and Greek Yogurt:

Ingredients:

- One medium apple
- One tsp of cinnamon
- Greek yogurt, two teaspoons (low-fat or non-fat)

Instructions:

- Set the oven's temperature to 175°C/350°F.

- After coring the apple, put it in a baking dish.

- Dredge the apple in cinnamon.

- Bake the apple for 20 to 25 minutes, or until it is tender.

- Top with Greek yogurt before serving.

- Savor your cozy and toasty dessert!

Nutritional Information (approximate):

- Calories: 153

- Protein: 5g

- Carbohydrates: 33g

- Fiber: 7g

- Fat: 2g

Cooking Suggestions and Grocery Lists for Your Metabolic Confusion Diet

Efficiently navigating the Metabolic Confusion Diet's precepts needs a thorough comprehension of not just its fundamental ideas, but also the savvy management of shopping purchases and culinary undertakings. In light of this, we provide a collection of culinary tactics and discriminating tips for efficient shopping purchases that are in sync with the Metabolic Confusion Diet:

Culinary Techniques:

- ***Preparatory Swiftness:*** It is advisable to set up a time each week for careful meal planning and culinary foresight. Slicing and slicing vegetables, marinating meats, and precooking staples like quinoa or brown rice might help to simplify times of culinary compulsion, imbuing temporal effectiveness.

- ***Communal Repast Production:*** It is practical to cultivate the practice of culinary mass production. Preparing large amounts of specialized meals that are malleable throughout many days is a powerful strategy. Consider arranging a large assemblage of grilled chicken or roasted veggies that lends adaptability to many culinary representations throughout the temporal domain.

- ***Select lean protein sources*** with caution, such as turkey, skinless fowl, lean beef cuts, fish, tofu, and tempeh. These substrates are required for the maintenance of lean muscle mass and the facilitation of metabolism.

- ***Embrace a variety of vivid veggies*** because they provide a symphony of diverse nutrients that promote overall vigor and metabolic balance.

- ***Assimilation of Beneficial Lipids:*** The incorporation of healthful fat sources—avocado, nuts, seeds, olive oil, and fatty fish—recommends itself. Such fats are necessary for the absorption of nutrients and the maintenance of hormonal balance.

- ***Aromatics Practice:*** Harness the power of herbs and spices as taste enhancers without resorting to excessive salt or sugary embellishment. Turmeric, cayenne pepper, cinnamon, and ginger, among others, not only tantalize the taste but also stimulate the metabolism.

- ***Complex Carbohydrate Incorporeality:*** Take advantage of the advantages of whole grains, such as quinoa, brown rice, whole wheat pasta, and oats. The abundance of these complex carbs provides long-term energy and fiber fortification.

- ***Exercising Prudence in Proportions:*** Exercising prudence in proportions is essential. Consuming excessive amounts, even of nutrient-dense elements, might have negative implications.

Grocery Shopping Guidelines:

Before beginning supermarket adventures, anticipate the weekly alimentary regimen via the architectonics of a precise meal stratagem. This strategy helps to avoid unnecessary purchases and supports smart resource usage.

Strategic Perimeter Sojourn: It is important to circumambulate the store's perimeter. This domain often includes a variety of fresh vegetables, lean meats, grains, and dairy—all of which are critical components of the Metabolic Confusion Diet.

Conscientious Protein Elicitation: Include a variety of lean protein options, such as skinless poultry, lean meat avatars, piscine entities, tofu, and leguminous versions.

Palettes Awash in Colorful Chromatics: Fill your basket with a diverse selection of veggies, whether fresh, frozen, or canned, that are free of unnecessary salt additives. A vibrant vegetal landscape indicates nutritional abundance.

Affirmation of Whole-Grain Dominion: Encourage the selection of whole grain emissaries like whole wheat bread, quinoa, brown rice, and whole wheat pasta that adhere to nutritional guidelines.

Eminence of Sapid Lipid Mediums: Encourage the incorporation of nutrient-rich lipids such as avocado, nuts, seeds, and olive oil, which go beyond culinary requirements to play the function of metabolic agents.

Herbal Embellishments: Compile a broad repertory of spices that promote metabolic stimulation, such as turmeric, cayenne pepper, and cinnamon.

Avoid Processed Comestibles: Avoid processed and saccharine-laden foods since their juxtaposition with the metabolic confusion ethos is incongruous.

Label Scrutiny: While speaking about packaged things, use caution when reading labels. Its scrutiny assures the absence of excessive carbohydrates, harmful fats, and severe salt augmentation.

Hydration Overture: Encourage hydration by bringing plenty of water and herbal infusions with you on your food trip.

Congruence with the Metabolic Confusion Diet is obtained by using these revered cooking tactics and prudent grocery preferences while engendering sustenance rich in nutrients. The intersection of consistency and balance is the foundation upon which the peak of health and fitness goals are accomplished.

Adjustments and plateaus: Listening to Your Body

Recognizing Your Body's Signals

Starting on the path of well-being needs an artistic understanding of the information your body sends. Through a variety of signs, your body, an excellent communicator, communicates its wishes, emotions, and moods. Let's go into the area of these signs, decoding your body's complicated language:

Hunger and Contentment:

- ***Gentle Grumblings:*** Your stomach's faint rumble or playful gnawing—your body's modest request for nutrition.
- ***Satiety:*** The feeling of completeness that comes with finishing a nice meal.

Fatigue and Energy Tides:

- ***The Lethargy Yawn:*** When exhaustion wraps about you like a comforting blanket, signifying the need for rest or renewal.
- ***Sparkling Vitality:*** The sensation of being energized, wide-eyed, and eager to grab the day—a symphony of energy harmonizing inside.

The Thirst Whispers:

- ***A dry tongue or a slight scratchiness***—the body's subtle warning to water, to drink from life's wellspring.

- ***The Call of Quenching:*** A thirst that calls, asking you to listen to your body's symphony of fluid requirements.

The Tango Digestif:

- ***Bloat's Murmur:*** A quiet belly bloom, a puff of discomfort—your body's request for a thoughtful encounter with digestion.
- ***The Digestion Dance:*** The ease of a well-executed tango, as shown by comfort and regularity in your belly motions.

Brushstrokes of Mood:

- ***The Tempest Within:*** An irritable tempest developing, clouds hiding the sun—a signpost for emotional rebalancing.
- ***The Sunlit Sky:*** A clean, serene emotional canvas splattered with serenity hues—a depiction of emotional balance.

The Symphony of Slumber:

- ***Tossing and tossing,*** sleep's illusive embrace—a midnight sonnet hinting at unfulfilled demands.
- ***The Dreamer's Oasis:*** Awakening refreshed, dreams woven in the fabric of slumber—a well-received nocturnal rhapsody.

Symphony of Cravings and Lullaby of Aversions:

- ***The crescendo of Cravings:*** A symphony of desire for certain tastes—a melody of the body's delicate yearnings.

- ***Whispers of Aversions:*** A faint refrain of revulsion, a pull away from particular flavors—a body's conversation in culinary preferences.

Physical Replicas:

- ***Headache's Echo:*** The throbbing rhythm of suffering, signaling the need for care and relief.
- ***Muscle's Sonata:*** The music of effort, a soothing reminder of your body's symphony in action.

The Skin Tapestry:

- ***Skin's Whisper:*** The dry caress or blemished stories your skin tells—a dermal-colored mural of well-being.
- ***Glowing Canvas:*** A glowing canvas with healthy skin—an artistic depiction of vitality inscribed on the body's parchment.

Heartbeat and Sigh of Breath:

- ***Accelerated Rhythms:*** A racing heart, a quickened pulse—possibly a song of effort or an echo of strain.
- ***Breath Unison:*** The rise and fall of breath, a cadence in peaceful synchronization—a breath symphony in peaceful concord.

Inner Thoughts:

- ***The Foggy Chronicles:*** Hazy thoughts, a mental labyrinth—a subtle prod toward attentive involvement.
- ***Clarity's Anthem:*** Crystalline thoughts, a mental vista—a victorious chorus of concentrated reflection.

The Weight Sonata:

The Ebb and Flow of Weight: The shifting melody of the scale—a rhythm tracing the cadence of living, presenting a chapter in your body's history.

By accepting these cues, you begin a path of attentive attention. Each cue, each murmur, creates a story in your body's language. By listening to your body's whispers, you create a harmonious relationship with its rhythm, choreographing a dance of health that resonates in the symphony of life.

Making Informed Changes to Your Approach

Any transformational journey, such as the Metabolic Confusion Diet, needs a dynamic strategy that adapts to your evolving requirements and objectives. Here, we provide a detailed and strategic strategy for making informed changes that not only correspond with your objectives but also cater to the complex interaction of your body and mind:

Consistent Self-Evaluation: Schedule time regularly to analyze your development and the efficacy of your present method.

- Investigate the details of your accomplishments as well as areas that need attention and development.
- Develop a keen awareness of how your body reacts to various stimuli, such as food modifications or exercise regimens.

Hone the skill of listening to your body's signs and signals, which frequently speak volumes about its demands.

- Develop awareness of minor changes in energy levels, mood patterns, digestion, and general health.
- Recognize when your body is expressing pain, exhaustion, or the need for restorative measures.

Data-Driven Progress Analysis: Make use of quantifiable data such as weight changes, body measurements, and fitness standards.

- Maintain detailed records that act as windows into your progress's tapestry, allowing you to discover patterns.
- Enlist the help of health specialists to appropriately assess these data points and derive important information.

Gradual Refinements: Make changes to your approach gradually to prevent sudden adjustments that might upset your balance.

- Observe your body's reaction to each change so that you can accurately estimate its influence.
- The progressive method allows for a more exact understanding of cause-and-effect dynamics.

Investigate Nutritional Insights: Keep a food diary or use digital applications to monitor your daily dietary intake.

- Analyze the macronutrient distribution—carbohydrates, proteins, and fats—to ensure that it corresponds to your body's specific needs.
- Adjust portion sizes, ratios, and meal scheduling based on your objectives for optimum nutrition.

Embrace Culinary Diversity: To avoid plateaus and maintain interest, include variation in your food and workout routines.

- Experiment with new meals, various training methods, and different food sources.
- This variety not only promotes physical improvement but also maintains your passion and drive.

Prioritize Recovery and Rest: Pay close attention to your body's recovery demands, providing enough time for recovery between strenuous exercises.

- Keep track of the quality and length of your sleep and adjust your routine to achieve maximum restoration.

- Recognize that appropriate healing and well-being are prerequisites for optimum growth.

Flexibility for Adaptation: Develop flexibility in your routines to account for changes in energy levels, daily responsibilities, and unexpected occurrences.

- Adapting to new situations smoothly eliminates interruptions and enables seamless integration of your method.

Periodic Reflective Assessment: Schedule extensive examinations of your growing plan to determine its effectiveness at regular intervals.

- Examine if your changes provide the desired results and identify areas for improvement.
- This iterative process of reflection ensures that your approach stays consistent with your ongoing experience.

Psychological Equilibrium: Recognize your journey's enormous influence on your psychological well-being.

- Be aware of pressures, emotional reactions, and mental resilience, while also acknowledging the interdependence of body and mind.
- Changes should include measures that promote a healthy balance of physical and emotional improvement.

Perpetual Learning and Growth: Develop a mindset of continual learning by being current on new research, trends, and holistic practices.

- Attend seminars, study credible sources, and engage in communities to broaden your knowledge.
- This dedication to knowledge guarantees that your modifications are well-informed and in line with the most recent findings.

Dealing with Plateaus: Breakthrough Strategies

On your journey to optimum well-being, conquering plateaus, those tough moments of stalled growth require subtlety and strategy. Here, we provide a toolset of smart techniques for breaking through plateaus and reviving progress, bringing you closer to your goals:

In-Depth Analysis and Correction:

- Examine your present routine holistically, including nutrition, exercise, and lifestyle choices.
- Identifying Stagnation: Determine where development has halted or become stagnant.
- Customized Tweaks: Tailor your changes to particularly target the regions that are exhibiting symptoms of stagnation.

Rethinking Your Routine:

- Spice up your workouts by changing up your training regimens to test different muscle groups and energy systems.

- Intensity and Length: Vary your exercise intensity, duration, and frequency to stimulate adaptation.

- Explore new activities, courses, or sports to revive your sense of adventure.

Rethinking Nutrition:

- Calorie Control: Adjust your calorie intake to fit your changing objectives and energy expenditure.

- Macronutrient Mastery: Tailor macronutrient ratios to your body's changing needs.

- Micro Boost: Make sure your body is getting the micronutrients it needs for best performance.

The Influence of Progressive Overload:

- Scaling Weights: Gradually increase weights, resistance, or intensity to keep your muscles challenged.

- Increasing Endurance: Gradually increase the time or intensity of your cardio exercises.

- Amplification of Skills: Improve your expertise and proficiency in your chosen pursuits.

Accept Periodization:

- Structured Stages: Divide your training into discrete phases, each with its own set of objectives and intensities.

- Alternate between high-intensity, low-volume periods and vice versa for cyclic mastery.

- Adaptation Prevention: By exposing your body to a variety of stimuli, you can keep it guessing and developing.

Putting Recovery First:

- Rest and Rejuvenation: Prioritize sleep, rest days, and relaxation for optimum healing.

- Lighter exercises such as yoga or mild stretches might help with active healing.

Mind-Muscle Interaction:

- Mindful Engagement: Focus your attention on the muscles you're working on during strength training.

- Form Finesse: Prioritize excellent form and coordinated motions rather than just lifting weights.

Stress Management:

- Stress-Relieving Strategies: Include stress-relieving techniques such as meditation, deep breathing, or mindfulness.

- Cortisol Management: Keep cortisol levels under control since chronically elevated cortisol might stymie improvement.

Community Strength:

- Accountability Allies: To keep on track, share your objectives with a buddy or join a group.
- Connecting with people going through similar experiences may bring support and insights.

Mental toughness:

- Resilience and Persistence: Recognize that plateaus are a normal part of any journey.
- Positive Attitude: Develop a development mindset by seeing setbacks as stepping stones to success.

Professional Advice:

- Seek assistance from experienced trainers, nutritionists, or healthcare specialists.
- New Points of View: Professionals may provide useful insights and personalized methods.

Goal Clarification:

- Reassess Ambitions: Consider if your objectives need to be adjusted depending on your success.

- Celebrating Victories: Acknowledge little victories along the road to boost your drive.

Beyond Diet, Sustainable Lifestyle Habits

Dietary choices are only a thread intertwined with countless other aspects that contribute to your overall vitality in the big tapestry of well-being. Embracing sustainable health extends beyond what's on your plate to include a symphony of activities that are in sync with your body, mind, and spirit. Let us go on a full examination of these multidimensional lifestyle behaviors that go well beyond diet:

1. Movement with Awareness:

- ***Diverse Physical Engagement:*** Participate in activities that appeal to you regularly, whether they be energizing runs, relaxing yoga sessions, dancing lessons, or team sports.

- ***Compassionate Consistency:*** Prioritize constant movement above intermittent bursts of intensity to cultivate a lifetime engagement with physical exercise.

- ***Take a Holistic Approach to Fitness:*** Combine cardiovascular activities for heart health with strength training to improve muscular integrity and general resilience.

2. Sleeping Well:

- ***Structured Sleep Routines:*** Create a consistent sleep plan to ensure you get 7-9 hours of refreshing slumber each night.

- ***Sleep Sanctuary:*** Create a sleep-friendly atmosphere by eliminating external distractions such as noise and light.

- ***Pre-Sleep Routines:*** To prepare your mind for sleep, develop peaceful nighttime rituals such as reading a book or practicing meditation.

3. Stress Control:

- ***Stress-Relieving Techniques:*** To counteract the effects of stress, participate in regular activities such as deep breathing, meditation, or mindfulness.

- ***Joy-Fueled Activities:*** Develop hobbies and activities that reflect your interests and provide a therapeutic outlet for stress relief.

- ***Work-Life Balance:*** Strive for a balance between work and personal life, avoiding chronic stress and promoting general well-being.

4. Rituals of Hydration:

- ***Hydrate Mindfully:*** Make constant water intake a priority throughout the day to support biological processes and keep hydrated.

- Increase your beverage repertoire by combining herbal teas and water infusions for a blast of flavor and added benefits.

- Listen to your body's thirst indicators and react quickly to maintain adequate water levels.

5. Relationship Nurturing:

- *Connection Promotes Well-Being:* Make time to cultivate meaningful connections, invest in shared experiences, and engage in open communication.

- *Empathy and Active Listening:* Foster emotional connections in encounters by practicing active listening and expressing empathy.
Recognize the importance of robust social networks in promoting emotional well-being, resilience, and a feeling of belonging.

6. Eating with Intention:

- *Attuned Nourishment:* Develop attentive eating habits by paying attention to hunger and satiety signals, savoring each meal, and enjoying the sensory experience.

- *Whole-Food Selections:* Choose nutrient-dense, whole foods that will fuel your body and give you sustained energy throughout the day.

- *Unplugged Eating:* Reduce distractions during meals so that you can completely interact with and appreciate your food.

7. Personal Development:

- *Setting Personal and Professional Objectives with Purpose:* Define personal and professional goals that match your interests, values, and development vision.

- *Lifelong Learning:* Encourage a sense of wonder by continually seeking out learning opportunities via books, seminars, or online courses.

- *Reflective Progression:* Take time to reflect on your path, appreciate your accomplishments, and re-align your objectives with your growing self.

8. Nourishing Mental Health:

- *Holistic Self-Care:* Prioritize self-care activities that are meaningful to you, such as spending time in nature, participating in hobbies, or practicing mindfulness.

- *Seek professional treatment* when necessary to address mental health difficulties and create healthy coping techniques.

- *Self-Image Empowerment:* Develop a good self-image by practicing self-compassion and accepting your individuality.

9. Retreats for Digital Detoxification:

- *Balanced Screen Time:* Set limits on screen time by designating tech-free intervals around meals and before sleep.

- *Immerse yourself in activities* that foster present-moment awareness, such as meditation, nature walks, or artistic endeavors.

- *Rekindle Genuine Connections:* Disconnecting from screens allows you to reconnect with yourself, others, and the environment around you.

10. Eco-Conscious Practices:

- *Reduce your ecological footprint* by adopting eco-friendly choices such as recycling, composting, and utilizing recyclable things.

- *Sustainable Mobility:* Choose environmentally friendly forms of mobility such as walking, cycling, or using public transportation.

- *Promoting Local and Organic Goods:* Prioritize local and organic products to help create a healthier earth and a more sustainable future.

11. Positive Resonance and Gratitude:

- *Daily Thanks Practice:* Set aside time each day to express gratitude for the blessings in your life, cultivating a feeling of happiness and abundance.

- *Constructive Optimism:* Develop a positive mindset by concentrating on solutions rather than problems.

- *Settings and Affirmations:* Create a positive atmosphere by including inspirational surroundings and uplifting affirmations.

12. Leisurely Rejuvenation:

- *Holistic Leisure:* Make time for things that offer you pleasure, relaxation, and a feeling of renewal.

- *Nurturing Hobbies:* Pursue hobbies and creative endeavors that feed your enthusiasm, encourage creativity, and provide an avenue for self-expression.

- *Balancing Act:* Balancing work and leisure responsibilities adds to overall life satisfaction and a happy living.

Conclusion

As we near the conclusion of our investigation into the Metabolic Confusion Diet for endomorph women and the larger world of long-term health, it's evident that the quest for well-being is a dynamic and nuanced path. Our journey has taken us through body types, metabolic techniques, hormonal complexities, nutrition, fitness, mental well-being, and lifestyle habits, exposing a complete tapestry that goes far beyond food issues.

Our adventure began with learning about the many landscapes of body types - ectomorphs, mesomorphs, and endomorphs - and how genetics impact our reactions to diet and activity. The Metabolic Confusion Diet emerges as a tailored method for endomorph women, using calorie variety, macronutrient cycling, and intermittent fasting to improve metabolism and stimulate development.

We've discussed the necessity of accepting uniqueness and forming a relationship with our bodies by delving into the realm of endomorph features, problems, and strengths. Unpacking the complicated dance between hormones and metabolic rates highlighted the critical significance of hormonal balance in overall well-being.

We've revealed the skill of maintaining metabolic dynamism and overcoming plateaus by navigating macronutrient cycling, caloric fluctuations, and their harmony with intermittent fasting. These tactics, when combined with specific training plans, such as exhilarating cardiovascular activity, provide a vivid image of a comprehensive fitness journey.

Beyond the physical, we've begun a psychological adventure, fighting cravings, navigating social environments, and monitoring progress. Recognizing the importance of meal preparation in long-term success, we've provided ourselves with the skills to make thoughtful decisions even in the middle of life's rush.

We've cherished the delights of culinary creativity via short, nutrient-dense meals, connecting nutritional sustenance with the larger mosaic of well-being. Furthermore, our story has walked supermarket aisles, read physical clues, explored intelligent adjustments, and embraced a balanced lifestyle that resonates deeply.

This journey has given me not just knowledge, but also a feeling of empowerment. You're equipped with information, techniques, and a bird's-eye perspective to confidently sail the ever-changing seas of well-being. Remember, this is your trip - a blank canvas waiting for your brushstrokes, the colors of your dreams, and the masterpiece of your life.

May you start on a lifetime journey of self-discovery, development, and nurture as you move ahead from these pages. Beyond food restrictions, you are called to live a life in which nutrition, exercise, mindfulness, relationships, and personal growth all work together to create a symphony of vibrant well-being.

With each chapter you write, each modification you create, and each milestone you reach, you become the architect of a tale that is uniquely yours - a story that is both amazing and gratifying.